You May Not Have
Irritable Bowel Syndrome

An Introduction to
Allergic Contact Enteritis
and the Food Allergies that Cause It

You May Not Have Irritable Bowel Syndrome

An Introduction to Allergic Contact Enteritis and the Food Allergies that Cause It

Michael Stierstorfer, M.D.
Medical Director,
IBS Centers for Advanced Food Allergy Testing

You May Not Have Irritable Bowel Syndrome:
An Introduction to Allergic Contact Enteritis and the Food Allergies that Cause It

Copyright © 2014 by Michael Stierstorfer, MD
IBS Centers for Advanced Food Allergy Testing

ISBN 978-0-692-34101-8

Cover Designers: RGA Communications
Medical Illustrator: Drew Strawbridge
Editor: Emily J. Weber

The names of all patients in this book have been changed.

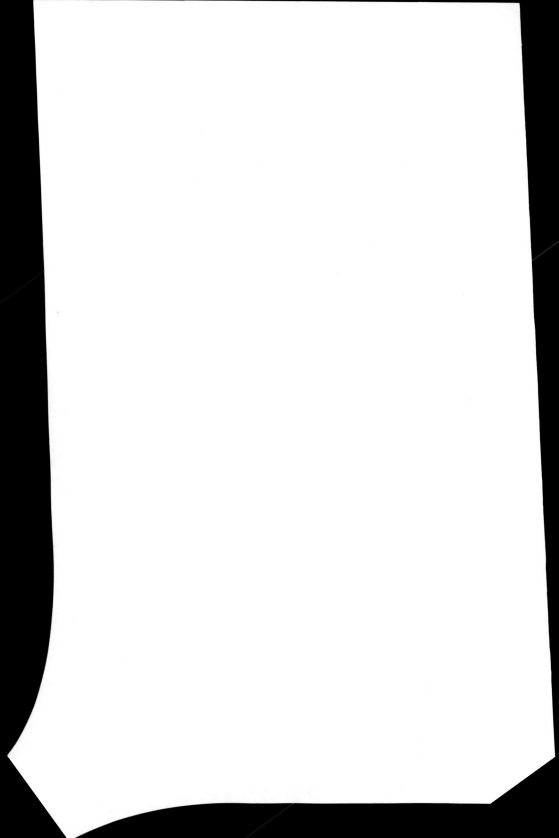

Dedication

This book is dedicated to my father, Max J. Stierstorfer, Jr., M.D., an old school general practitioner whose office was in the home where I grew up. Fourteen-hour work days and house calls were routine, as were the delivery of babies and the occasional removal of tonsils in the early days. Countless patients have told me they always felt better when they left his office than when they came in. He was a pillar in his community, a master diagnostician, a Navy veteran, a tireless advocate for the disadvantaged, an outspoken proponent of tort reform, a trailblazer in sports medicine and healthcare cost containment, and an inspiration to all who knew him.

Contents

PREFACE xiii

CHAPTER ONE: OVERVIEW.............................. 15
    The Big Issues 15
    What's the Big Deal?................................... 16
    Course of the Disease 16
    Quality of Life... 17
    Economic Cost 17

CHAPTER TWO: SO WHAT'S NORMAL? 19

CHAPTER THREE: MAKING A DIAGNOSIS 21
    Associated Medical Conditions 22

CHAPTER FOUR: WHAT'S THE CAUSE? 25
    Current Theories 25

CHAPTER FIVE: EVALUATION 27

CHAPTER SIX: TREATMENT OVERVIEW 31
    Diet.. 31
    Mental Health Therapy.............................. 34
    Medication 35

CHAPTER SEVEN: THE PATH TO DISCOVERY 45
    A Game-Changing Observation 45
    The Case That Spawned the Discovery 46
    Proof-of-Concept Study.............................. 49

CHAPTER EIGHT: PULLING IT ALL TOGETHER 55

CHAPTER NINE: WHO MAY BENEFIT FROM
FOOD PATCH TESTING? 61

CHAPTER TEN: THE STATE OF THE ART 63

BIBLIOGRAPHY 74

ABOUT THE AUTHOR 87

Acknowledgements

I am grateful to the following people for their efforts with my research on the subject matter and preparation of this book: Leslie Heffron, Sally Iles, Phyllis Stierstorfer, Ryan Elias, Ph.D., John Floros, Ph.D., Marvin Sasson, M.D., Chris Sha, M.D., Anton de Groot, M.D., Ph.D., Harry Mansfield, Julie Campion, Mark Taylor, Phil Bennett, Mark Pimsley, Christine Maginnis, Joel Gelfand, M.D., Bruce Brod, M.D., Johnny Im, Drew Strawbridge, Bob Borghese, Steve Krawet, M.D., Amy Levinson, C.R.N.P., Kris Mitlas, Olivia Petrovich, Carol Smith, Keri Davis, Krista Ammon, Judy Weber, Emily Weber, and Brent Barnett.

Preface

If you have irritable bowel syndrome (IBS), you're not alone. An estimated 32 to 48 million Americans and many more worldwide have it, or think they have it as defined by the criteria used to make the diagnosis. It's no fun: the discomfort itself, the uncertainty as to what's going on and where it will lead, the recognition that it's often a lifelong problem, the interference with work and leisure activities, not to mention the burden of always having your belly on your mind. I'm happy to report there is hope. An identifiable cause and potential cure for many IBS sufferers has been discovered. In fact, as the title of this book suggests, you may not have IBS at all. You may have a newly discovered disease: allergic contact enteritis (ACE).

This book will provide an overview of IBS as it is currently understood; look at its impact on society; define IBS and describe how the diagnosis is made; present theories regarding contributing factors; outline a multitude of treatment options; and dispel some common myths along the way. It will present groundbreaking insights into the cause of IBS that have led to the recognition of and testing for this new disease, allergic contact enteritis, that can help and in many cases cure people who carry a diagnosis of "IBS." Finally, it will introduce the state-of-the-art IBS Centers for Advanced Food Allergy Testing, whose sole mission is to help individuals pinpoint unique specific food allergies that are causing their IBS symptoms.

If I had been told years ago when graduating from medical school or four years later when I completed my specialty training in dermatology that one day I'd be writing a book about IBS, I wouldn't have believed it. But here I am—not only writing a book but also introducing this discovery that may be one of the biggest advances in the understanding and treatment of IBS since the disease was first described in the 1950s. How did this come to be?

As fate would have it, when I was confronted with the onset of what seemed for all the world like IBS, I was perfectly positioned as a dermatologist to make some simple observations, use a little common sense and deductive reasoning, and take advantage of a time-tested tool in dermatology, skin patch testing, to identify a unique type of food allergy that likely was causing my symptoms. Also using my training and position as a dermatologist, I was subsequently able to design and carry out a clinical study that suggested the same type of food allergy was causing IBS symptoms in others. Chapter Seven and beyond will provide a step-by-step account of the discovery process and support for the theory. My own experience and the subsequent proof-of-concept study lend credence to this newly identified disease that mimics IBS, which I have descriptively named allergic contact enteritis (ACE). My newfound interest in IBS and the ability to help people who suffer from it have been an extremely rewarding addition to my life's work, the practice of dermatology.

If you are knowledgeable about IBS, you already may be familiar with much of the information in Chapters One through Six, in which case you may want to skip right to Chapter Seven, where the description of the revolutionary discovery of ACE begins.

If you are not yet knowledgeable about IBS, Chapters One through Six will cover much of what has been known about it up to the time of this discovery and the myriad of treatment options.

Chapter One

Overview

The Big Issues

In reviewing the medical literature, three major issues are included in most everything written about irritable bowel syndrome (IBS). First, IBS is referred to as a "functional" disease; in other words, one in which there is nothing physically wrong with the gastrointestinal (GI) tract. Second, it always is referred to as a disease for which the cause is unknown. Third, there are many different treatment approaches to IBS, none of which is effective in all cases, and many that are not very effective at all.

As a result of my discovery which came from supporting evidence from the clinical study we performed and the testing we currently offer IBS patients, there is now an answer for all three of these problematic issues for many people suffering from IBS or, as you will see, what was once thought to be IBS.

A recent national survey on IBS patient educational needs identified several additional questions of great interest:

- Are there certain foods I should avoid?
- What coping strategies are recommended?
- Will I have IBS the rest of my life?
- What medications are available?
- What is the current research?
- How do psychological factors affect IBS?
- What is "normal bowel habit"?[1]

This book will answer all these questions including, for the first time, a definitive cause and potential cure in many cases. If you have IBS and have tried everything there is to try without relief, don't be discouraged—help may well be on the way. This chapter and the next five chapters provide an overview of the heretofore "state of the art" of IBS. There are many theories about IBS that offer partial explanations for how IBS behaves, but until now, there has been no unifying theory. You will see how this new theory elegantly pieces together many of the previous observations, culminating in what is now understood as allergic contact enteritis.

What's the Big Deal?

IBS affects between 10 and 15 percent of people in Western countries[2, 3] and many more worldwide. It is about twice as common in women as it is men in the United States and Europe[4] but is of about equal incidence in Africa, southern Asia and South America.[5] It is most common in those between twenty-five and fifty-four years of age.[4]

More than three out of four individuals with IBS in the United States do not know what they have or haven't been given an "official" diagnosis, and only about 25 percent of IBS sufferers are under professional health care.[6]

Course of the Disease

IBS is a chronic condition with 16 percent reporting diagnosis within the past year, 8 percent in the previous one to two years, 26 percent in the previous two to five years, 14 percent in the previous six to ten years, and 33 percent reporting the condition for more than ten years. Symptoms remain fairly constant over the entire course of the disease: 73 percent reported the condition being stable long-term, while just 22 percent reported some improvement over the years.

IBS sufferers experience symptoms on average 8.1 days per month with abdominal pain and discomfort being the most common symptom.[4] On symptomatic days, patients experience symptoms on average more than twice a day, with over half of the episodes lasting longer than sixty minutes.[4]

Quality of Life

Patient complaints relating to "functional" bowel disorders are often trivialized,[7] but IBS has about the same impact on quality of life as other common chronic diseases such as asthma and migraines.[8] A recently published collection of in-depth interviews has revealed details about its impact. About 25 percent of IBS patients report missing social functions due to their IBS.[4] Taking long trips and vacations and dining out are reported to be more of a problem for IBS sufferers vs. non-IBS sufferers. Many feel they need to be near a toilet or make frequent trips to the restroom. IBS sufferers also have more difficulty making new friends and having physical relationships than those without it. A number of IBS sufferers feel their condition affects family relationships. About 25 percent of IBS sufferers report diminished self-confidence.[4]

Economic Cost

IBS is a major burden to the economy as well. Loss of work productivity, the chronicity of the disease, a lack of effective treatment for many, and health care costs all contribute to the economic burden.[9]

About 3.5 million visits to physicians in the United States each year are for irritable bowel syndrome, making up about 25 percent of all patients seen in gastroenterologists' practices.[10] IBS is the seventh most common diagnosis made by all physicians and the most common made by gastroenterologists.[10]

Despite these numbers, only about 25 percent of all individuals with IBS symptoms seek medical care.[11, 12, 13] One report showed current IBS sufferers saw a doctor an average of 4.2 times in the last twelve months if they had been medically diagnosed but just 1.3 times if they had not been medically diagnosed.[4]

IBS accounts for $1.6 billion in medical costs in the U.S. annually.[14] Direct health care costs per individual with IBS in the United States range from $742 to $3,166 per year, significantly higher than in individuals who do not have IBS.[15] Additionally, indirect costs due to lost work productivity total an estimated $19.2 billion a year in the United States.[15] Absenteeism from work in individuals with IBS is more than twice that of non-sufferers (6.4 vs. 3.0 days)[1]. One in six IBS sufferers change his or her work schedule, and one in four work fewer hours.[1] While at work, 67 percent of IBS sufferers feel less productive due to difficulty with concentration and time management.[4]

Chapter Two

So What's Normal?

Since IBS characteristically involves a change in bowel habits, understanding what's normal is important. The better question is: What's normal for you? If you are feeling well and you have not experienced a consistent change in your pattern of bowel movements (frequency, shape, consistency), then that's probably normal for you, even if it's not considered "average" for others.[16]

"Average" is one or two bowel movements a day. Some go more often, while others go as infrequently as once a week. If you go just once or twice a week but don't have to strain, that can be normal for you. Three or fewer bowel movements a week with the need to strain defines constipation. Fewer bowel movements than one a week should increase the level of concern.[16]

Shape can vary; pencil-thin stools, while sometimes indicating a problem, can also be normal. Watery diarrhea is abnormal.[16]

Color can also vary. Brown is normal. Black tarry stools can indicate blood in the stool, but black stools also may occur when taking iron supplements or bismuth subsalicylate. Color change to gray clay can indicate a block in the flow of bile or liver disease. Red may indicate GI bleeding, but beetroot red is normal after eating beetroots.[16]

The Bristol Stool Scale grades stool shape and consistency on a scale from 1 to 7 (see Appendix 1[17]). Types 3, 4 and 5 are considered normal. Types 1 and 2 are typical of constipation, while Types 6 and 7 indicate diarrhea.[17]

Chapter Three

Making a Diagnosis

First and foremost, evaluation by a qualified healthcare provider is essential. The diagnosis of IBS is made based on symptoms.[1] A physical examination is essential to help rule out other conditions, but there is nothing in a physical exam nor any diagnostic tests that can confirm a diagnosis of IBS. Symptom-based criteria called the Rome III criteria, published in 2006, are most commonly used to diagnose IBS.[18] These criteria are summarized here:

Abdominal pain or discomfort at least three days per month during the previous three months, accompanied by at least two of the following:

1. Relieved by having a bowel movement;
2. Onset associated with a change in stool frequency, either constipation or diarrhea (when bowel movements become more often or less often);
3. Onset associated with a change in stool form or appearance (when the stools are getting harder or softer).

Other accompanying symptoms that would give further support to a diagnosis of IBS include the following: [19]

1. Change in how you move your bowels (straining and/or urgency)
2. Clear or white mucus in the stool
3. Abdominal bloating or a feeling of distension
4. Heartburn
5. Early feeling of fullness when eating
6. Nausea
7. Upper abdominal discomfort that comes and goes
8. The feeling of incomplete emptying

For example, if you have had belly discomfort for six days last month and three days each of the previous two months, and you find that you feel better after a bowel movement, and the onset of your symptoms was accompanied by your stools becoming harder, then you would qualify for a diagnosis of IBS, assuming you had no "red flags" (see Chapter Five).

By comparison, if you had belly pain three or more days each of the past three months, and your pain was relieved by moving your bowels but there was no change in stool hardness or softness and no diarrhea or constipation, then you would not be considered to have IBS as defined by the Rome III criteria.

The diagnosis can be challenging, as suggested by the fact that in one survey, 25 percent of those who were diagnosed with IBS had visited a health care professional five or more times before the diagnosis was made.

IBS is classified as constipation- (IBS-C) or diarrhea-(IBS-D) predominant, or alternating between the two (IBS-A).[19] About a third of IBS sufferers fall into each category. Treatment options, which will be presented in Chapter Six, typically are determined at least in part by the category into which the individual falls.

Associated Medical Conditions

As is the case with many diseases with no known cause, there are many misconceptions about IBS. These include that it can cause malnutrition or cancer, that it is caused by lack of digestive enzymes, that it is a form of inflammatory bowel disease (IBD) such as Crohn's disease or ulcerative colitis or can develop into IBD, or that it usually will worsen with age. All are false.[1] Despite the significant negative impact on quality of life, IBS is not associated with other serious physical illness.

Not surprisingly, given the disruptive symptoms of IBS, psychological issues are common, including anxiety, depression, and neurosis.[20] One study showed a higher incidence of suicidal thoughts and attempts due to IBS.[7] IBS is also more common in patients with other functional disorders, such as fibromyalgia and chronic fatigue.[21] It is this author's opinion that oftentimes these psychological problems, fibromyalgia, and chronic fatigue may be a consequence of suffering with the chronic symptoms of IBS rather than its cause.

Chapter Four

What's the Cause? (Pre-ACE Discovery)

In short, prior to the discovery of allergic contact enteritis, the cause of IBS has been unknown. That doesn't mean there aren't a lot of sensible explanations based on observations of IBS that have been made over the years. Unfortunately, none of these explanations has resulted in treatments that have cured IBS. Treatments certainly may help, but after they are stopped, the symptoms will almost always reliably recur.

Current Theories

Altered bacteria in the gastrointestinal tract: Using a lactulose hydrogen breath test, a study published in 2000 showed that 78 percent of IBS patients tested had bacterial overgrowth in the small intestine. Nearly half improved after antibiotic treatment eliminated the overgrowth.[22]

Immune dysregulation: A 2002 study showed evidence of inflammation in the lining of the intestine of IBS patients.[23]

Increased intestinal permeability: A 2004 study showed that individuals with IBS more easily absorb lactulose, a disaccharide sugar that isn't normally well absorbed from the GI tract.[24]

Alterations in GI serotonergic transmission: Serotonin is a natural chemical messenger that stimulates intestinal motility, which is the contraction of muscles that propels contents in the GI tract. A 2006 publication reported individuals with diarrhea-predominant IBS have higher levels of the natural chemical messenger serotonin, and those with constipation-predominant IBS have lowered serotonin levels in the bloodstream.[25]

Abnormal GI motility: Specific abnormalities of large and small bowel motility have been observed and are associated with symptoms in IBS, as reported in 1991.[26]

Visceral hypersensitivity: A 2002 report suggested the nervous system of some people with IBS seems to be more sensitive to stimuli such as intestinal distension.[27]

Post-infectious bowel changes: In 2006, a study showed that IBS sometimes will first appear after gastrointestinal infection.[28]

Psychological factors: Chronic stress is believed to contribute to IBS. Chronic stress can lead to overactivity of the sympathetic nervous system, the part of nervous system that helps us adapt to stress. The sympathetic nervous system also plays a role in normal GI functioning, so its overactivity may contribute to IBS symptoms.[29]

Central processing of pain perception: As reported in 2002, some people with IBS are hypervigilant to stimuli, resulting in greater perception of pain.[27]

Genetic factors: Heredity also may play a role. A 2003 report questioned whether this is due to true genetic susceptibility or a learned illness behavior.[30]

It is generally accepted that a single cause is unlikely to be responsible for all cases of IBS. Rather, more than one factor likely contributes in any given case.[31] Treatment directed at each factor helps some IBS sufferers, suggesting that each factor plays a role in some cases.

Chapter Five

Evaluation

The diagnosis of IBS can be made on clinical grounds alone. A thorough medical history and physical examination performed by a qualified medical practitioner should be enough to make the diagnosis. If the information you provide to your health care provider about the history of your condition meets the Rome III criteria previously presented, and if there are no warning signs or symptoms of other GI diseases based on your history or physical exam, then the diagnosis of IBS can be made with confidence. There is no need for extensive laboratory testing or other diagnostic tests such as GI procedures or radiographic imaging studies.

Despite this, a large proportion of patients with symptoms of IBS are referred to specialists for consultation to rule out other diseases or to confirm the diagnosis of IBS. Motivation for such referrals may include the reassurance of a second opinion for the patient and/or primary care provider, so that another diagnosis is not overlooked. These referrals often result in unnecessary tests and, rarely, surgery being performed.[32, 33, 34]

Signs and symptoms, referred to as "red flags," that may suggest more dangerous conditions include: sudden onset, loss of appetite, weight loss, symptoms causing awakening from sleep, gradually worsening symptoms, onset at age fifty or older, blood in the stool, fever, painless diarrhea, rectal bleeding, gluten intolerance, fat in the stool, and iron deficiency anemia.[19] Laboratory and radiologic testing for patients younger than fifty who fit the diagnostic criteria for IBS and have no "red flags" are not recommended[34], with the exception of a family history of

Crohn's disease, ulcerative colitis, celiac disease or colorectal cancer, which could legitimately prompt further diagnostic testing.

For individuals with some of the red flags, screening laboratory tests include both stool and blood studies. Stool studies include examination for ova and parasites in search of conditions such as tapeworm; disease-causing bacteria; white blood cells, presence of which is suggestive of gastrointestinal infection; *Clostridium difficile* toxin (*C. difficile* are bacteria normally present in the large intestine in small numbers which can overgrow and cause serious illness when other normally present bacteria are killed by antibiotics); and giardia antigen (giardia is a parasite infection from ingestion of contaminated food, soil or water). Blood work includes a complete blood count with differential to look for evidence of infection, anemia or inflammation, as well as a comprehensive metabolic profile to look for dehydration and electrolyte imbalances in individuals with diarrhea and to evaluate for metabolic disorders.

Other studies are guided by historical clues. They include hydrogen breath testing (see Sidebar 1) to screen for lactose intolerance, fructose intolerance, and bacterial overgrowth; and blood tests to screen for thyroid or parathyroid problems and inflammation.[19] Depending on the "red flag," diagnostic imaging studies such as upper GI with small bowel follow through or CT scan, or GI studies such as upper and/or lower endoscopy may be warranted.

Additionally, some authorities recommend that everyone who meets the diagnostic criteria for IBS be screened for celiac disease, which can mimic IBS.[35] Screening tests for celiac disease include a blood test for transglutaminase antibody and small bowel biopsy.

Sidebar 1: The Hydrogen Breath Test

The hydrogen breath test is used to diagnose sugar malabsorption or small intestine bacterial overgrowth (SIBO), both of which may be present in IBS. The only source of hydrogen in the human body is via metabolism of sugars by bacteria in the gastrointestinal tract. Normally, very little hydrogen is produced because most sugar is absorbed from the small intestine into the bloodstream, before it reaches the large intestine where most bacteria reside. When not properly absorbed, sugars reach the large intestine where they are available for bacterial fermentation and formation of hydrogen.

Likewise, in SIBO, the bacterial population migrates into the small intestine, where they have access to the sugars. When exposed to bacteria in the intestine, sugar is metabolized to hydrogen, which is quickly absorbed into the bloodstream, exhaled, and measurable in expired air. Thus, an elevated level of hydrogen as measured by the hydrogen breath test is an indirect measure of sugar malabsorption or small intestine bacterial overgrowth.[42]

Still other available diagnostic testing falls in the realm of alternative medicine. Such studies include serum IgG levels to food antigens,[36] salivary IgA,[37, 38] intestinal permeability studies,[39] and fecal short chain fatty acid level measurements.[40] These studies are yet to be proven effective by rigorous study in making diagnosis and treatment decisions.[41]

Chapter Six

Treatment Overview (Pre-ACE Discovery)

Generally in the field of medicine, the more ways to treat a disease, the harder it is to treat. Irritable bowel syndrome is no exception. What follows is an encyclopedic listing of many of the available treatments, grouped by the aspect of IBS toward which they are directed. None of the old established treatments can be expected to cure IBS because you can't cure something if you don't know what's causing it. Rather, most treatments have been directed at symptoms, some at underlying contributing factors.

Often combinations of treatments are used. Once these treatments are stopped, symptoms will reliably recur in the great majority of cases. Instead, the therapeutic goal has been a reduction in the frequency and severity of symptoms and a general improvement in the quality of life.

Diet

The prevalence of IBS has increased over the past fifty years in countries where a Western-style diet has been more prominent.[4] The majority of people with IBS believe that certain foods trigger their IBS symptoms,[4] but most are unable to identify the specific foods responsible. Dietary strategies are a central part of most treatment regimens. Dietary management generally takes a tiered approach, starting with simple measures and progressing to more complex dietary management depending on one's response to simpler measures.

First-line dietary measures: The simplest measures address lactose, a natural sugar found in milk, and dairy products, and general advice about dietary fiber (non-starch polysaccharides).

Many people lack the enzyme lactase and are unable to properly digest lactose. This trait is most common in those of Mediterranean, Asian, Native American, African and South American descent. Undigested lactose results in gas, bloating, belly pain and diarrhea, the same symptoms often experienced in IBS. Avoidance of lactose ingestion will help at least the significant percentage of IBS sufferers who happen to be deficient in the lactase enzyme.

Gradual introduction of oral fiber supplementation is widely recommended for IBS, but its beneficial effect is not well established. There are two types of dietary fiber: soluble and insoluble. Over-the-counter soluble fiber includes polycarbophil compounds (Citrucel®, FiberCon®) and psyllium compounds (Metamucil®). Soluble fiber acts as a bulking agent, and for many IBS-D patients, allows for a more consistent stool. For IBS-C patients, it seems to allow for a softer, moister, more easily passable stool. Soluble fiber seems to benefit 30 to 50 percent of IBS recipients.[43]

Insoluble fiber such as corn and wheat bran[19] may help ease constipation,[44] but may cause bloating and abdominal distension in some people with IBS.[45] Legumes such as beans, lentils, peas, peanuts and chickpeas, which also are high in insoluble fiber, may contribute to bloating and generally should be limited in the diet.[19]

Also common is intolerance to the monosaccharide sugars sorbitol, fructose, and xylitol, and to caffeine, and their avoidance should be tried as part of the first-line dietary measures.[43]

Second-line dietary measures (FODMAP Diet): Fermentable carbohydrates are not digested or absorbed well in the intestine and thus can be fermented by bacteria, producing methane and hydrogen. They draw water into the gastrointestinal tract and cause symptoms of bloating, gas, cramping and/or diarrhea in some individuals with IBS. A diet low in fermentable carbohydrates, called a FODMAP diet,[46] is recommended if simpler dietary measures fail. FODMAP stands for Fermentable Oligo-Di-Monosaccharides and Polyols.[47]

FODMAPs include the following foods:[47]
1. Fructose: high fructose corn syrup, honey and fruits
2. Lactose: dairy
3. Fructans: onion, garlic and wheat
4. Galactans: beans, lentils and legumes such as soy
5. Polyols: sugar alcohols such as sorbitol and mannitol; stone fruits such as avocado, peaches, nectarines, plums, cherries, and apricots; and sweeteners containing sorbitol, xylitol, mannitol, and maltitol.[47] Sugar-free chewing gum is a major source of sorbitol.[46]

Exclusion of foods high in fermentable carbohydrates is recommended for four to eight weeks and indefinitely if helpful in relieving symptoms. Up to 70 percent of IBS patients benefit from FODMAP diets.[46]

Probiotics:[48] Probiotics are live microorganisms, mostly bacteria, which provide a health benefit when administered in adequate amounts. The balance of "good" and "bad" bacteria in the GI tract in patients with IBS is different than in healthy people[49] and has been the rationale to use probiotics in IBS treatment to restore the balance. In one study, 68 percent of individuals taking probiotics vs. 37.5 percent taking a placebo experienced relief of IBS symptoms after four weeks of treatment.[48] Studies have shown that probiotic supplementation contributes to improvement of gut motility,[48] reduction in inflammation[49] and reduction in visceral hypersensitivity,[50] all of which may help alleviate IBS symptoms. A trial of at least four weeks is advised.

Third-line dietary measures: An elimination diet may be tried when a specific food seems to trigger IBS symptoms. A two- to four-week trial is recommended.[45]

Mental Health Therapy[31, 51, 52]

Emotional stress does not cause IBS but can make symptoms worse. The gut in many people with IBS seems more sensitive to stress, so taking lifestyle advice and learning techniques to cope with stress is a central part of most treatment regimens.

Simple ways to reduce stress for most everyone include regular sleep and exercise and finding enjoyable hobbies, good friendships, and other pleasurable activities.

Psychotherapy may be helpful, especially for those with IBS that is severe or responds poorly to treatment and those with more prominent psychosocial issues.

The various types of therapy, alone or in combination, include:

Cognitive therapy: The basic premise is that thoughts influence moods. By working on identifying and evaluating automatic negative thoughts about themselves, the world, and/or the future, people can think more realistically and thus feel better emotionally and behave more functionally.

Behavioral therapy: Behavioral therapy is a treatment that helps change potentially self-destructive behaviors and replaces bad habits with good ones.
Psychodynamic therapy: Directed at interpersonal problems, it helps people understand the causes of emotional distress and focuses on how emotions affect IBS symptoms.

Educational Therapy: This therapy is used to treat individuals with learning differences and disabilities and to help strengthen their ability to learn. Efforts focus on academics as well as teaching the processing of information, focusing, and memory skills.

Hypnotherapy: The power of suggestion is more effective when the person is in a hypnotic state and can help relax the muscles of the colon. It can also be used to search for a possible psychological root cause of a symptom, such as a traumatic past event that a person has suppressed.

Medication

Some IBS sufferers will be fortunate and benefit from some combination of the dietary changes and mental health therapy. Many, however, will not and may require medications in search of some relief. Choice of medications may be tailored to the specific symptoms of any given individual and typically is directed at gastrointestinal motor or gastrointestinal sensory symptoms, or central nervous system processing.[51] It may take some trial and error to find a medication that works well. Unfortunately, most medical treatments are often not particularly effective, and their beneficial effects may be short-lived. To worsen matters, many have troublesome side effects and none are curative.

Medication for irritable bowel syndrome should start with measures to reduce symptoms related to constipation and diarrhea. Often in patients with constipation-predominant IBS, regular passage of stool will reduce pain and bloating. In patients with diarrhea-predominant IBS, its treatment can improve quality of life by decreasing stool urgency and frequency but usually does not reduce pain.[51]

This review will include medications available only in the United States.

Note: Rx=prescription; OTC=over-the-counter

Symptom: Diarrhea

Medications prescribed to treat diarrhea include:

- **Loperamide**[51] (Imodium®), Rx and OTC
- **Bismuth subsalicylate** (Kaopectate®, Pepto-Bismol®), OTC
  These medications may be used to improve stool frequency and consistency but are not useful in treating abdominal pain, bloating or other IBS symptoms. They should be used in the lowest dose that helps.

- **Cholestyramine** (Questran®, Questran Light®, Prevalite®, Locholest®), Rx
  Cholestyramine is a bile-acid binder, which may be added to control diarrhea poorly responsive to other treatment. A nighttime dose of a bile-acid binder is often very effective in patients with diarrhea-predominant irritable bowel syndrome who have had their gall bladder removed.[53]

Symptoms: Diarrhea and Pain

Antispasmodics: "Spastic colon" is another name for IBS. Anticholinergic agents, opioid agonists, and serotonin antagonists all may serve as antispasmodics. They can provide short-term relief of abdominal pain and discomfort of IBS by relaxing muscles in the stomach and intestine. In practice, they are taken 30 minutes before meals to reduce urgency and cramps after meals. Fast-acting sublingual and long-acting antispasmodic agents are available. Additionally, they slow transit time and allow the intestines to draw moisture out at a normal or higher rate and help stop the formation of loose and liquid stools.[51, 54]

Anticholinergics prescribed to treat diarrhea and pain include:

- **Dicyclomine** (Bentyl®), Rx
- **Hyoscyamine** (Levsin®, Anaspaz®, Levbid®), Rx
  These medications are taken as needed before meals that are expected to cause cramping. Common, typically mild and readily-reversible side effects include dry mouth, blurred vision, fatigue, and urinary hesitancy. They should not be used in individuals with narrow-angle glaucoma or urinary retention. Because of their safety, low cost, and utility given on an as needed basis, these drugs are generally tried first if more conservative measures have failed.[51, 55]

- **Phenobarbital/hyoscyamine/atropine/scopolamine** (Donnatal®), Rx
- **Chlordiazepoxide/clidinium bromide** (Librax®), Rx
- **Belladonna/butabarbital** (Butibel®), Rx
  These formulations combine barbiturate or benzodiazepine sedatives with anticholinergic medications and are best reserved for severe IBS flares when anticholinergic agents alone have failed. Addiction risk is low given intolerable anticholinergic side effects at higher doses.[51]

- **Peppermint oil,** OTC
  Peppermint oil is a natural antispasmodic that may be effective in relieving pain and diarrhea. It is cheap, safe, and readily available. Enteric coated capsules are recommended, as peppermint may aggravate heartburn.[56]

Opioid Agonists: [19, 51, 57]

Opioid agonists prescribed to treat diarrhea and pain include:

- **Diphenoxylate/atropine** (Lomotil®), Rx
- **Diphenoxin/atropine** (Mototofen®), Rx
  Lomotil® and Motofen® contain the opioid agonists diphenoxylate and diphenoxin, respectively, and also a very low dose of atropine which helps slow gut movement. Lomotil® and Motofen® could have opioid-like effects if taken in excess, and atropine could have intolerable side effects at higher doses, so its presence also minimizes the potential for misuse of these medications. Although unlikely, physical and mental withdrawal symptoms from both anticholinergic rebound caused by atropine and opiate withdrawal caused by difenoxin or diphenoxylate are possible if taken for long periods of time.

Serotonin Antagonists: Serotonin is a natural hormone that stimulates GI motility.[58] These medications block the effect of serotonin and thereby slow down gut motility.

Serotonin antagonists prescribed to treat diarrhea and pain include:

- **Alosetron** (Lotronex®), Rx[19, 59]
  Alosetron is an FDA-approved serotonin antagonist for women with severe IBS whose main symptom is diarrhea. Because it can cause rare serious side effects, including ischemic colitis and severe constipation, Alosetron is only used if other medicines do not work. Alosetron is not approved for use in men.

Symptom: Constipation

If fiber supplements such as psyllium, methylcellulose, and polycarbophil do not help relieve constipation, medication should be considered.

Osmotic Laxatives: [52, 60] These medications work by drawing water into the GI tract. The FDA has warned that taking more than one dose of sodium phosphate in twenty-four hours can cause rare but serious harm to the kidneys and heart, and even death due to severe dehydration and electrolyte imbalances.

Osmotic laxatives prescribed to treat constipation include:

- **Polyethylene glycol** (MiraLax®), OTC
- **Magnesium citrate** (Citroma®), OTC
- **Magnesium hydroxide** (Phillips Milk of Magnesia®), OTC
- **Magnesium sulfate,** OTC
- **Docusate sodium** (Colace®), OTC
- **Sodium phosphate,** OTC
- **Potassium sodium tartrate,** OTC
- **Lactulose,** Rx
- **Sorbitol,** OTC

The last two listed, lactulose and sorbitol, are non-absorbed carbohydrate laxatives and are effective but expensive and can result in the formation of gas and bloating discomfort.[52]

Stimulant Cathartics: These medications are more likely than other laxatives to cause cramping. They can become less effective over time and are associated with dependency. They are not recommended for long-term use.[51]

Stimulant cathartics prescribed to treat constipation include:

- **Senna** (Senokot®), OTC
- **Bisacodyl** (Dulcolax®, Fleet®, Correctol®), OTC

Chloride channel activators: Chloride channel activators increase fluid secretion into the lumen of the GI tract, leading to softening of the stool and increased intestinal motility. The available chloride channel activator is approved for female patients with IBS-C. Its effectiveness in men has not been proven. Common side effects include nausea, diarrhea, and abdominal pain.

The chloride channel activator prescribed to treat constipation in women is:

- **Lubriprostone** (Amitiza®), [61] Rx

Guanylate cyclase agonist: The medication in this class recently has been approved for moderate to severe IBS-C and acts by elevating cyclic guanosine monophosphate (cGMP) levels, leading to accelerated gastrointestinal transit through increased fluid secretion and reduced visceral hypersensitivity, i.e. reduced pain.[62]

The guanylate cyclase agonist prescribed to treat constipation is:

- **Linaclotide** (Linzess®, Constella®), Rx

Symptom: Diarrhea or Constipation

Tricyclic antidepressants: [51, 52, 63, 64, 65] Tricyclic antidepressants are recommended for the treatment of moderate to severe IBS when abdominal pain is a major issue or when other treatments have failed. They can be used in combination with antispasmodic agents if either treatment alone has been partially helpful. Their effect could be due to a reduction in the sensitivity of peripheral nerves or to alterations in the brain, but not due to their antidepressant effects. Lower doses than are needed to treat depression are effective for IBS. Their anticholinergic effects are responsible for their side effects, including constipation, slowing of urine flow, dry mouth, blurred vision and sleepiness. Narrow angle glaucoma and urinary retention are contraindications. Slowing of GI transit may be of therapeutic advantage in diarrhea-predominant IBS (IBS-D), but this class of medications also may be helpful for constipation-predominant IBS (IBS-C). They should be taken before bed due to the potential for sedation.

Tricyclic antidepressants prescribed to treat diarrhea or constipation include:

- **Imipramine** (Tofranil®), Rx
- **Amitryptaline** (Elavil®), Rx
- **Doxepin** (Sinequan®), Rx
- **Desipramine** (Norpramin®), Rx

Serotonin re-uptake inhibitors (SSRIs): These medications prevent reuptake of serotonin, act to stimulate GI motility, and can be particularly helpful in IBS-C, especially when accompanied by a mood disorder or if tricyclic antidepressants have failed. They lack the side effects but generally are not as effective as tricyclic antidepressants.

Serotonin re-uptake inhibitors prescribed to treat diarrhea or constipation include:

- **Fluoxetine** (Prozac®), Rx
- **Citalopram** (Celexa®), Rx
- **Paroxetine** (Paxil®), Rx

Antibiotics: [66, 67, 68, 69] As previously mentioned, findings suggest that patients with IBS have excessive bacteria in the small intestine, known as bacterial overgrowth. This overgrowth of bacteria can cause excessive gas production with a variety of non-specific symptoms such as diarrhea, bloating, abdominal pain and constipation. A short-term course of non-absorbable antibiotics is a newer treatment option, helpful in reducing diarrhea, constipation, abdominal pain and bloating in IBS. These antibiotics are poorly absorbed from the GI tract into the bloodstream and thus have very low side effect risk and have an effect only on bacteria located within the small and/or large intestine.

Antibiotics prescribed to treat diarrhea or constipation include:

- **Rifaximin** (Xifaxan®), Rx
  A two week course of rifaximin has been shown to maintain symptom relief in patients with IBS for more than three months after treatment is discontinued.

- **Neomycin,** Rx
  Neomycin has been used in similar circumstances as rifaximin, but because development of bacterial resistance is common, it is typically used only in combination with rifaximin for IBS sufferers with a methane-positive lactulose breath test. This combination of both antibiotics is more effective than either antibiotic alone in this circumstance.

Symptom: Pain

Medications prescribed to treat pain include:

- **Pregabalin** (Lyrica®), Rx
- **Gabapentin** (Neurontin®), Rx
  These drugs modify pain receptors and may help manage IBS-related abdominal pain.[70]
- **Chinese herbal mixtures**[51, 52]
  There have been no good studies confirming their effectiveness. Differences in purity and ingredients complicate evaluation.

Treatment Summary

As you can see, there are many IBS treatment options. The varying degree of treatment success, the often transient nature of the benefit, and the "trial and error" approach to treatment that is frequently taken can be equally frustrating for patients and their physicians. A recent survey showed that more than 45 percent of patients with IBS were not satisfied with any of their available treatment and management options.[71, 72] This dissatisfaction rate appears to be higher than that of other chronic diseases such as migraine headaches, depression and chronic constipation. One poll showed 46 percent of IBS sufferers agreed they would "try anything" to relieve their IBS symptoms.[4]

The key is to try to identify a cause for these symptoms which, until now, has never been done in most cases. In my dermatology practice a similar situation often arises when I am confronted with patients who are on several medications and develop a typical "measles-like" drug rash. As I explain to them, I can give them prescription creams and anti-itch pills that may help relieve their symptoms to some degree, but until we figure out which medication is causing their rash and stop it, they won't get much better.

Placebo effect is the effect that a treatment that is not "real" may have on a medical condition. IBS is known to have a high rate of responsiveness (between 30 and 40 percent) to placebo treatment. Evaluation of treatment effectiveness must take this into account.[73]

Chapter Seven

Necessity is the mother of invention.

English proverb

The Path to Discovery

A Game-Changing Observation

An extremely important step in figuring out the root cause of IBS is a relatively recent observation that inflammation is present in the gastrointestinal tract of people with IBS. This is crucial since it refutes previous theories that IBS is a "functional" disease. By definition, the fact that there is inflammation means there is something physically wrong; it's not "functional". Inflammation has been shown to affect motility of the GI tract, and altered motility has been shown to cause IBS symptoms. Finally there is observable evidence of something physical—inflammation—that can cause IBS symptoms.[74, 75, 76, 77, 78]

Direct evidence of inflammation comes from a landmark study revealing inflammation and nerve damage in biopsies taken from the small intestine in patients with severe irritable bowel syndrome. The biopsies showed white blood cells called lymphocytes within the intestinal wall and around nerves in the intestinal wall. The presence of white blood cells is a major feature of inflammation. The nerve damage observed in the majority of these biopsies is likely caused by the inflammation.[74]

Indirect evidence of inflammation comes from two observations. First, patients with inactive inflammatory bowel disease have a higher than expected incidence of IBS, which may be due to continued mild inflammation.[79, 80] Additionally, some cases of IBS have been known to start after bouts with bacterial or viral gastroenteritis, suggesting that inflammation may be at the root of IBS.[81]

That brings us to the biggest question of all: *What causes the inflammation?* Since most people with IBS have not had inflammatory bowel disease or recent infectious gastroenteritis, there must be another explanation for the inflammation in most cases.

The Case That Spawned the Discovery

As is true with many major advances in medicine, this groundbreaking discovery was not rocket science, and as mentioned in this book's preface, it was spawned by my own misfortune or good fortune, depending how you look at it. I will present with some degree of detail the case—my own—that fostered my interest in IBS so that you can follow the thought process behind the discovery and, as we later were able to show, behind what is likely the cause for IBS symptoms in many people. The best part? It is beautifully simple and will appeal to those of you who are fans of common sense.

At age forty-eight, in otherwise excellent health, out of the blue I developed a mild bellyache and bloating sensation and later additional symptoms typically associated with IBS. At first, I thought it was from something I ate at a rather suspect Mexican restaurant earlier that day. I assumed it would go away by the next morning. It didn't. Instead, the symptoms persisted with varying severity about half of my waking hours. Gluten and lactose avoidance did not help.

After three months, I qualified as having IBS since I met the diagnostic criteria outlined in Chapter Three, despite not yet having sought medical care. These symptoms lasted for a year. I finally sought evaluation by a gastroenterologist who performed an extensive work up including upper and lower endoscopic exams, an upper GI with small bowel follow through barium x-ray study, an abdominal and pelvic CAT scan, a hydrogen breath test and several laboratory tests. Two studies showed slow motility of the small intestine but nothing else.

This evaluation was quite time consuming and disruptive to my work. It ended up costing my medical insurance carrier about $7,500 and exposed me to the risk of anesthesia and significant radiation. Nevertheless, I was happy to pursue all this testing as I was eager to find out what was wrong.

Shortly after completion of the evaluation, I ate at two Indian restaurants within a week and both times experienced severe flares of the IBS symptoms, convincing me it had to be something in the food I had just eaten. Prior to that, I couldn't find any definite correlation with food. I thought long and hard about what was in that Indian food that I could be eating regularly in other foods as well. While I didn't eat Indian spices frequently, I realized that the one ingredient in most Indian food that is in many foods most of us eat all the time in the average American diet is garlic. So I avoided garlic, and within a day or two, my IBS symptoms completely disappeared. After that, if I accidentally ate something with garlic in it, I would reliably develop the same symptoms within an hour or two, and they would resolve again within a day.

At that point, I asked myself: Is this an intolerance or an allergy to garlic? I reasoned that it would be unusual at age forty-eight to suddenly become intolerant to garlic. A new allergy would be more likely. Importantly, an allergic reaction doesn't necessarily have to be to something new. It can be to something you've eaten your entire life, and your immune system just decides at some point to become allergic to it.

There are four types of allergies, types 1 through 4. Types 1 and 4 are the most common and the easiest for which to test. Type 1 allergies cause hives, seasonal allergies, and asthma and can result in anaphylaxis from foods like peanuts. Type 1 allergies are routinely evaluated by allergists with prick and scratch testing and a blood test called a RAST test, which measures specific IgE antibodies. I ordered an IgE RAST test on myself to garlic, and the result was negative. In reviewing the medical literature, I subsequently learned that type 1 allergy testing has been found not helpful in the evaluation of IBS. A landmark report in 2010 by the National Institutes of Health on *all* aspects of food allergy makes no mention of the use of type 1 allergy testing for IBS[82] despite the fact that it is common practice to do so among some health care providers. So while food allergies appear to be involved, as you'll see shortly, testing for type 1 allergies in IBS is like barking up the wrong tree—looking for the wrong type of allergy.

The type of allergy for which dermatologists frequently test is the type that causes a skin rash called **allergic contact dermatitis**, which is a form of eczema. Poison ivy is perhaps the most well-known example of allergic contact dermatitis. This is called a type 4 allergy. Dermatologists often test for type 4 allergies when evaluating patients with eczema if we are suspicious that their eczema may be due to an allergic reaction to something touching their skin.

The test we use is a tried-and-true test in dermatology called a patch test (see Appendix 2). It is a simple, painless, non-invasive test in which the substances in question, called allergens, are placed in contact with the skin on the patient's upper back. Strips of tape containing small wells, called patch test strips, are used to affix and cover the allergens on the back—thus the name "patch tests." The patches are removed from the skin after forty-eight hours, and the back is then examined to see whether any of the areas of skin in contact with the allergens are inflamed—typically a small red mark. Sometimes the skin's response doesn't occur until a day or two after removing the patches, so the patient returns again a day or two later for one final patch test reading. The testing should not be done on patients taking medications that suppress the immune system since they may prevent the skin from developing an allergic response (i.e., a positive patch test), which could result in an allergy being missed.

I applied a small slice of garlic to my skin, removed it forty-eight hours later, and a remarkable thing happened—a small itchy red spot had developed under the patch, indicating a type 4 allergy. With these results in mind, I reasoned that if my skin was reacting to contact with garlic, then there was no reason that the lining of my gastrointestinal tract couldn't do the same thing when food containing garlic was passing through. After all, the immune system has as much access to the lining of the GI tract as it does the surface of the skin, maybe more. This allergic reaction in the GI tract likely was causing inflammation that could affect the motility and cause the IBS symptoms.

Proof-of-Concept Study

In researching IBS further, to my surprise I found that this type of food allergy testing had never been investigated for IBS. It seemed unlikely to me that I would be the only person in the world to develop IBS symptoms and find evidence—the positive patch test to garlic—suggesting it was the result of a type 4 food allergy. I hypothesized that many people with IBS experience the same thing; namely, they have a type 4 allergic reaction along the lining of the intestine to the same type of foods that are known to cause type 4 allergic reactions on the skin, just like in my case. So if type 4 allergies cause IBS symptoms, then the most likely culprit foods to use in skin patch testing on people with IBS should be foods known to cause type 4 allergic skin reactions. For reasons previously mentioned, foods that typically cause type 1 allergies (peanuts, shellfish, etc.) would *not* be appropriate candidates for this testing.

To investigate this hypothesis, my dermatology practice performed a clinical study for individuals with IBS or IBS-like symptoms, testing up to forty foods all known to cause type 4 allergies. We were able to pinpoint a food allergy in some participants and were unable to do so in others. Independent of their own results, most study participants provided feedback that they were grateful we were doing this investigation because nothing was helping them.

Thirty out of fifty-one study patients had a positive patch test to at least one food. Those with a positive patch test then avoided the foods in question for one week. Fourteen of the fifty-one (more than 27 percent) improved—three slightly, eight moderately, and three greatly. The most common food to which people were allergic and benefited from avoiding was garlic, so I wasn't alone in my issue with garlic (see Sidebar 2).

Sidebar 2: The "Next Gluten"?

It's interesting that about 70 percent of IBS patients improve on a low FODMAP diet (see Chapter Six). Perhaps they improve for the reasons suggested in Chapter Six, but did you notice that garlic avoidance is part of this diet? In our clinical study, garlic was by far the most commonly identified type 4 food allergen. Seven of the fourteen patients who benefited in our study were allergic to garlic. Perhaps many of those benefiting from the FODMAP diet are allergic to garlic and benefit because this diet includes garlic avoidance. Could many people walking around with what they believe to be IBS actually have ACE caused by garlic ingestion?

Could garlic be "the next gluten" in terms of the impact of a single food on gastrointestinal health? Further investigation is needed.

Of the study patients who benefited, eleven reported back to me more than three months later, and ten of the eleven maintained their improvement, weighing against a placebo effect. The only one who didn't maintain her improvement experienced only mild improvement in the study and reported she didn't eat much sodium benzoate, which is a preservative to which she reacted with the patch test.

To summarize, we have found that type 4 food allergy patch testing can precisely identify specific foods that, when removed from the diet of people with IBS or symptoms suggestive of IBS, improves or completely cures their IBS symptoms. Our study, Food Patch Testing for Irritable Bowel Syndrome, was published in March 2013 in the Journal of the American Academy of Dermatology.[83]

These results support the hypothesis that many people who carry a diagnosis of IBS actually have a type 4 food allergy, which I have descriptively named **allergic contact enteritis**, or ACE for short. The enteric nervous system is the part of the nervous system that supplies the gastrointestinal tract.

To translate in non-medical terms: *ACE is an **allergic** reaction resulting from **contact** of the lining of the GI tract with food to which a type 4 allergy has developed, resulting in **enteritis*** (i.e., inflammation of the part of the nervous system that supplies the gastrointestinal tract) and causing IBS-like symptoms (see Sidebar 3). This hypothesis and the results of our study may spark a number of questions, some of which will be addressed in the next chapter.

Sidebar 3: Culinary Adventures

Discovering the garlic allergy has resulted in quite an adventure for me. Since garlic is in many processed and ethnic foods, the allergy has forced me to alter my eating habits. Now I read food labels carefully. If the ingredient list includes "spices" or "natural flavors" and I'm unable to check with the manufacturer, I stay away from them since garlic could fall under either category. I have found that restaurants that can best accommodate this allergy are also the ones that cook from scratch and tend to be the better restaurants anyway. When I start feeling sorry for myself because I can't eat pepperoni pizza, I get over it quickly when I remember what it felt like to walk around with an upset stomach half the time. Fortunately, I have found that the tomato sauce on New York style pizza tends to be garlic-free!

It's been an ongoing learning process. I underwent testing to the 120 food allergens we now have available (see Chapter Ten). In addition to garlic, my skin tested positive to allyl isothiocyanate, which comes from mustard seed. After learning of the mustard allergy, I realized in retrospect that on the rare occasions I ingested mustard I would often develop an upset stomach, which would go away by the next day. The part of garlic responsible for allergies is a chemical structure known as an "allyl group," so it is not surprising that I react to another food containing an allyl group, allyl isothiocyanate, as well. Mustard is not nearly as common as garlic in the foods Americans typically eat, so for me mustard caused only an occasional upset stomach since I ate it infrequently. It is likely that if I ate it as often as I did the ubiquitous garlic, I would develop frequent enough symptoms to qualify for a diagnosis of IBS.

I subsequently tested myself to well-cooked garlic, and my skin did not react. Cooking garlic apparently alters its chemical structure so that it becomes less likely to cause an allergic reaction the longer it is cooked. Predictably, I can eat well-cooked garlic without developing IBS symptoms, although I don't try it too often since I don't always know how well the garlic is cooked and don't want to risk ruining my day. I recently challenged myself with the best Italian-crafted sandwich you will ever find from a hole-in-the-wall restaurant near the sports arena complex in South Philadelphia. One ingredient is garlic that has been roasted for a long time. I enjoyed two sandwiches with no belly issues afterwards!

Garlic is a member of the plant genus *Allium*. Luckily for me, I can eat most other vegetables in the *Allium* genus—onions, shallots, chives, leeks—without consequence, but I found that after frequently eating large quantities of scallions (also in the *Allium* genus) over the course of a month in my two favorite garlic-free Chinese and Korean dishes, the same IBS symptoms developed. It finally dawned on me what I was doing. I stopped eating the scallions and was fine. As you might predict by now, a subsequent patch test to scallion showed a positive reaction.

Each of these observations lends support to the theory presented.

Chapter Eight

Pulling It All Together

Near the beginning of this book, three big IBS issues were identified: its prevailing "functional" nature (i.e., there's nothing physically wrong), its unknown cause, and the multitude of treatment options. At long last, there is a likely answer for these issues in many people, and the answer is that for those whom the food patch testing helps, it's not IBS after all—it's allergic contact enteritis (ACE).

The key is the recent evidence of inflammation in the lining of the gastrointestinal tract in people with IBS. So IBS is not a "functional" disorder. **It's not in your head. There is something physically wrong.**

For a small percentage of people, the inflammation is due to coexistent inactive inflammatory bowel disease. For another small percentage, it is post-infectious gastroenteritis. What about the rest—the large majority of IBS sufferers who never had inflammatory bowel disease or infectious gastroenteritis? For the first time since IBS has been recognized as a distinct condition, we have identified what appears to be the cause in many and a contributing factor in many others, and it all makes perfect sense: Type 4 food allergies cause inflammation along the lining of the intestine. The inflammation in turn affects the nerves that control motility in the GI tract. The altered motility may speed up or slow down food passage. Speeding up the motility may cause diarrhea and abdominal discomfort, perhaps due to spasm; slowing things down causes constipation and allows for bacterial overgrowth and bloating due to gas build up.

Either way, allergic contact enteritis (ACE) mimics the symptoms of IBS. All the treatments previously listed help some part of this process, but none cure it. Eliminate ingestion of the food or foods identified by skin patch testing and, for many, the symptoms improve or resolve completely.

This new theory and new disease may raise some questions for which I offer these possible answers:

What about IBS sufferers who do not benefit from any of the existing treatments or from food patch testing?
Their symptoms may have some other cause yet to be discovered, or perhaps they may have type 4 allergies to other foods for which they were not tested.

Why did those with IBS for which type 4 food skin allergies were identified in the clinical study not benefit from avoidance of those foods in their diet?
Perhaps they did not follow the avoidance diet adequately; perhaps there are other foods to which the person is also allergic but were not tested and are still being eaten; perhaps there is not always a direct correlation between the amount of inflammation in the skin from patch testing and the amount of inflammation along the GI tract from the food passing through; or perhaps different people have different thresholds for developing GI symptoms from the inflammation that develops along their intestinal lining.

Why doesn't everyone who demonstrates a type 4 skin reaction from patch testing develop full-blown IBS from eating the same foods?
As in my case with mustard, perhaps they don't eat the food in question and have the symptoms frequently enough to qualify as having "full-blown" IBS. As previously mentioned, I have a type 4 skin reaction to allyl isothiocyanate, which is found in mustard seed, and I develop abdominal discomfort after eating mustard.

But because I ate mustard so infrequently, the symptoms would go away within a day and wouldn't come back until I ate mustard again quite later. They didn't occur often enough to meet the diagnostic criteria of IBS.

Why do the GI symptoms reported here begin an hour or so after ingesting garlic, while skin rashes and symptoms of allergic contact dermatitis like poison ivy usually don't appear until a day or two after contact with the allergen?
The answer, I believe, is that the top dead layer of skin, the stratum corneum, provides a protective barrier through which it takes allergens extra time to pass before they gain access to the immune system, stationed deeper in the skin. It is the interaction between the offending allergen and the immune system that results in the inflammation and the itchy rash known as allergic contact dermatitis (see Appendix 3), as seen with positive food patch tests. Unlike the skin, the lining of the GI tract has no such protective layer, so food allergens have much more direct access to the immune system positioned in the wall of the GI tract (see Appendix 4).

Likewise, why do GI symptoms often resolve within a day or two after avoiding the food in question? After all, poison ivy takes two or three weeks to go away if not treated.
I believe the answer is that the lining of the GI tract renews much faster than skin (four days for the GI tract vs. twenty-eight days for skin), so the inflammation in the GI tract also likely clears up much more quickly.

Why don't symptoms occur in the upper part of the GI tract from these allergies?
They actually can, resulting in inflammation and symptoms of the lips (allergic contact cheilitis[84]) and mouth (allergic contact stomatitis[84]). The same thing likely occurs in the esophagus

(eosinophilic esophagitis) and stomach (eosinophilic gastritis). Probably because food passes through these parts relatively quickly and has longer contact time with the lower GI tract (i.e., the small and large intestine), the immune response and consequent symptoms tend to develop in the lower GI tract instead.

The FODMAP diet does not implicate allergies or account for the inflammation observed in IBS, yet it is effective in a large percentage of IBS sufferers who try it. How does this tie in with type 4 food allergies?

At least for some, it is likely that allergic reactions to type 4 food allergens alter motility of the GI tract, making FODMAP carbohydrates more accessible to the bacteria that ferment them and produce the hydrogen and methane that contribute to IBS symptoms. For those for whom a type 4 allergy is found to play a role, it seems likely that the FODMAP diet reduces hydrogen and methane that contribute to IBS symptoms, but avoidance of the type 4 food allergen removes the true root cause of the problem. One thing is certain: if one or two type 4 food allergens that are responsible for someone's IBS symptoms can be identified by patch testing, their avoidance would generally be much easier than trying to follow the FODMAP diet.

Is food patch testing worth it for everyone with IBS symptoms?

In our current healthcare environment, any new treatment intervention for IBS should be evaluated for effectiveness and economic viability, especially in light of the huge impact of IBS on our quality of life and on our economy.[85] Our experience at the IBS Centers for Advanced Food Allergy Testing (see Chapter Ten) has been that the testing services are covered by some insurers, and as recognition of the value of this new testing grows, more insurers will be eager to make it readily available for their customers. In the absence of insurance coverage, the relatively modest costs of food patch testing compared to the costs associated with an extensive evaluation such as mine (see Chapter Seven) warrant its consideration as *a cost-effective, first-line intervention for IBS sufferers not responding to conservative measures.*

Chapter Nine

Who May Benefit From Food Patch Testing?

For starters, **the 32 to 48 million Americans and countless others worldwide who suffer from IBS are all good candidates**. The testing won't provide an answer for everyone, but if it helps almost 50 percent, including the approximately 20 percent who are cured, numbers based on our current experience (see Chapter Ten), that would put a significant dent in the world's suffering and costs due to IBS. Of utmost importance is the need for a qualified healthcare provider to be sure there are no "red flags" (see Chapter Five) suggesting other GI conditions before pursuing patch testing.

As mentioned, **those with just an occasional upset stomach** for a day or two for no good reason may benefit. If the food to which the individual is allergic is eaten infrequently, it could still result in GI distress, even though symptoms may not meet the criteria used to diagnosis IBS. A type 4 food allergy could be responsible and detectable by the patch testing.

We have tested patients who believed they had IBS who developed consistently pencil-thin stools a few years before developing their belly pain. Pencil-thin stools may be a warning sign of colon cancer and should always be evaluated by a healthcare provider. If colon cancer is ruled out, patch testing could detect a food allergy responsible for **change in stool shape**. After specific food allergies were identified in our patients and the foods were avoided, the stool form returned to normal.

Likewise, some of our patients reported being "gassy" for years prior to developing their full-blown IBS. After identifying type 4 food allergies via the patch testing, our patients with this issue often reported their "gassiness" went away with avoidance of the foods in question, so it is likely that **excessive flatulence** is another good reason to consider the food patch testing.

As mentioned in Chapter Eight, type 4 food allergies are known to cause inflammation of the lips (**allergic contact cheilitis**[84]) and mouth (**allergic contact stomatitis**[84]). Additionally, there are two rarer GI conditions, **eosinophilic esophagitis**[86, 87] and **eosinophilic gastroenteritis**,[82] for which food allergy is suspected, but testing with type 4 food allergens has not been investigated. While we have no experience using our patch testing for these conditions, all should be good candidates for the testing.

Leaky gut syndrome is a condition generally not accepted in mainstream medicine. Its believers feel that there may be a connection between leaky gut and some diseases such as diabetes, lupus, multiple sclerosis, and even autism. The theory is that the small intestine in leaky gut syndrome is more permeable than normal, allowing toxins, microorganisms, undigested food or waste to leak through into the bloodstream, which activates immune responses that contribute to various disease states.[88, 89, 90] The cause of the "leakiness" is not known. Could inflammation from type 4 food allergies be the cause of a leaky gut? I do not know the answer to this question, but it may warrant further investigation if leaky gut syndrome gains stronger scientific support.

Chapter Ten

The State of the Art

As previously mentioned, the work presented here would be considered in the scientific community "proof-of-concept" work. Proof-of-concept work typically involves a small pilot study to investigate whether there is any merit to a new concept and to determine whether it may be worthwhile to pursue a larger, more rigorously designed study that might statistically validate the concept. We are collecting data and making other efforts to perform such validation work.

In the meantime, rather than withholding this testing from those who potentially could greatly benefit, we have developed, with the help of licensed compounding pharmacists and university-based food scientists, an extensive panel of food allergens for patch testing now available at the **IBS Centers for Advanced Food Allergy Testing**. We have assembled 120 foods and food additives for the testing (see Appendix 5). They include all kinds of commonly consumed foods such as vegetables, artificial flavors, emulsifiers, binders, thickeners, and preservatives. Importantly, they are all foods known to cause type 4 allergies, not foods like peanuts and shellfish that typically cause type 1 allergies.

Our centers are dedicated solely to the performance of food patch testing for people with IBS, symptoms suggestive of IBS, and the other GI conditions described in Chapter Nine to investigate whether type 4 food allergies may be playing a role. All other aspects of care are referred back to the primary care provider and/or gastroenterologist. It should be noted that, like much patch testing performed in the United States for the evaluation of skin rashes, the food patch testing for IBS is not FDA-approved. The food allergens are imported from reputable patch test manufacturers in Canada and Germany or are prepared in the

United States by licensed compounding pharmacists, using only high-grade edible food components in standardized formulations.

Currently, we help almost half of the people with IBS whom we test, including about twenty percent whom we've cured (see Sidebar 4). If food allergies are identified, we provide information on how to avoid the specific food or foods and recommend not eating them for one month. If the patient notices improvement in his or her IBS symptoms, then he or she is advised to avoid the food or foods indefinitely, because once you have an allergy, it usually doesn't go away. You likely have a friend for life!

Sidebar 4: Case Studies

With our current testing, we recently have cured people previously believed to have IBS by identifying allergies as diverse as benzoyl peroxide (used to bleach flour) and cinnamon.

Some other representative examples of patients who have benefited from this testing:

- Donna, a fifty-year-old woman had a positive patch test to limonene, which is found in citrus. She reported she drank tea with lemon every night. When she stopped adding lemon to her tea, her IBS went away.
- Sarah, a twenty-three-year-old woman with a strong patch test reaction to nickel saw significant improvement with a low nickel diet, which is an extremely difficult diet to follow (see Appendix 6).

The flagship IBS Center for Advanced Food Allergy Testing is located in Philadelphia, Pennsylvania, with plans to open other centers around the country. More information about the testing and location of test centers is available online at **www.IBSfoodallergy.com** and on the YouTube video **Food Patch Testing for Irritable Bowel Syndrome**.

Bristol Stool Scale

Type 1		Separate hard lumps, hard to pass
Type 2		Sausage-shaped but lumpy
Type 3		Like a sausage but with cracks on surface
Type 4		Snake-like, smooth and soft
Type 5		Soft blobs with clear cut edges, pass easily
Type 6		Ragged edges, mushy stool
Type 7		Watery diarrhea

The Bristol Stool Scale was developed by K. W. Heaton and S. J. Lewis at the University of Bristol and first published in the Scandinavian Journal of Gastroenterology in 1997.[17]

Patch Testing

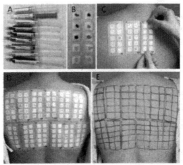

A Food allergens in standard patch test formulations
B Food allergens on patch test strips
C Patch test strips being applied to skin
D All 120 food allergens applied to skin
E All patches removed 48 hours later and back
  marked for patch test reading

Patch Testing

Typical positive patch test
(actual size is about 1/3 inch)

Skin

Microscopic View Cross Section

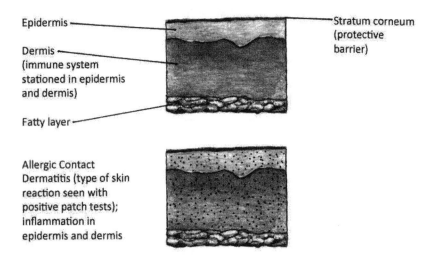

Epidermis

Dermis
(immune system
stationed in epidermis
and dermis)

Fatty layer

Stratum corneum
(protective
barrier)

Allergic Contact
Dermatitis (type of skin
reaction seen with
positive patch tests);
inflammation in
epidermis and dermis

Intestine
Microscopic View Cross Section

Mucosa

Submucosa
(immune system
stationed in mucosa
and submucosa)

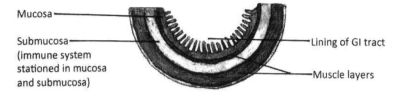

Lining of GI tract

Muscle layers

Allergic Contact
Enteritis, theoretical
cause of IBS symptoms
(note similarity to
Allergic Contact
Dermatitis in skin-
Appendix 4)

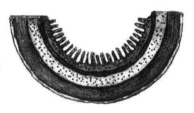

Appendix 5
Food Allergens for Patch Testing*

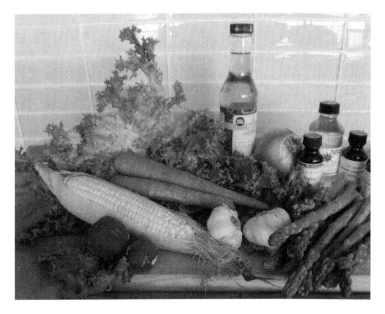

*Representative examples

Low Nickel Diet

Permitted Foods
All meats
Poultry
Fish (except Herring)
Eggs
Milk
Yogurt
Butter
Cheese
Potatoes (1 medium-sized per day)
Small amounts of the following:
    Cauliflower
    Cabbage
    Cucumber
    Lettuce
Polished rice
Flour (except whole grain)
Fresh fruits (except pears)
Marmalade/jam
Coffee
Wine Beer

Prohibited Foods
Canned foods
Acid foods cooked in
    stainless steel utensils
Herring
Oysters
AsparagusBeans
Mushrooms
Onions
Corn
Spinach
Tomatoes
Peas
Whole grain flour
Fresh and cooked pears
Rhubarb
Tea
Cocoa and chocolate
Baking powder
Margarine
Mayonnaise

Bibliography

1   Halpert A, Dalton CB, Palsson O, Morris C, Hu Y, Bangdiwala S, Hankins J, Norton N, Drossman D. What patients know about irritable bowel syndrome (IBS) and what they would like to know. National survey on patient educational needs in IBS and development and validation of the patient educational. Am J Gastroenterol 2007:102(9):1972-1982.

2   Camilleri M, Choi MG. Review article: irritable bowel syndrome. Aliment Pharmacol Ther 1997; 11:3-15.

3   Talley NJ. Irritable bowel syndrome: definition, diagnosis and epidemiology. Ballieres Best Pract Res Clin Gastroenterol 1999; 13:371-384.

4   Hungin APS, Chang L, Locke GR, Dennis EH, Barghout V. Irritable bowel syndrome in the United States: prevalence, symptom patterns and impact. Aliment Pharmacol Ther 2005; 21(11):1365-1375

5   Lovell RM, Ford AC. Effect of gender on prevalence of irritable bowel syndrome in the community: systematic review and meta-analysis. Am J Gastroenterol 2012; 107:991-1000.

6   Luscombe FA. Health-related quality of life and associated psychosocial factors in irritable bowel syndrome: a review. Qual Life Res 2000; 9:161-176.

7   Miller V, Hopkins L, Whorwell PJ. Suicidal ideation in patients with irritable bowel syndrome. Clin Gastroenterol Hepatol 2004; 2(12):1064-1068.

8   Frank L, Kleinman L, Rentz A, Ciesla G, Kim JJ, Zacker C. Health-related quality of life associated with irritable bowel

syndrome: comparison with other chronic diseases. Clin Ther 2002; 24:675-689.

9 Davis RH. Overcoming barriers in irritable bowel syndrome with constipation (IBS-C). J Fam Pract 2009; 58:S3-7.

10 Everhart JE, Renault PF. Irritable bowel syndrome in office-based practice in the United States. Gastroenterology 1991; 100:998-1005.

11 Camilleri M, Williams DE. Economic burden of irritable bowel syndrome. Proposed strategies to control expenditures. Pharmacoeconomics 2000; 17(4):331-338.

12 Talley NJ, Zinsmeister AR, Melton LJ 3rd. Irritable bowel syndrome in a community: system subgroups, risk factors, and health care utilization. Am J Epidemiol 1995; 142:76-83.

13 Camilleri M. Management of the irritable bowel syndrome. Gastroenterology 2001; 120(3):652-668.

14 Drossman DA, Camilleri M, Mayer EA, Whitehead WE. AGA technical review on irritable bowel syndrome. Gastroenterology. 2002; 123:2108-2131.

15 Martin BC, Ganguly R, Pannicker S, Frech F, Barghout, V. Utilization patterns and net direct medical cost to Medicaid of irritable bowel syndrome. Curr Med Res Opin 2003; 19(8):771-780.

16 Bharucha AD, Seide BM, Zinsmeister AR, Melton III LJ. Insights into normal and disordered bowel habits from bowel diaries. Am J Gastroenterol 2008; 103(3):692-698.

17   Heaton KW, Lewis SJ. Stool form scale as a useful guide to intestinal transit time. Scandinavian Journal of Gastroenterology 1997; 32(9):920-924.

18   Longstreth GF, Thompson WG, Chey WD, Houghton LA, Mearin F, Spiller RC. Functional bowel disorders. Gastroenterology. 2006; 130(5):1480-1491.

19   Lehrer JK, Lichtenstein GR. Irritable Bowel Syndrome. emedicine.medscape [Internet]. [Cited 2014 May 22]; Available from: http://emedicine.medscape.com/article/180389-overview.

20   Solmaz M, Kavuk I, Sayar K. Psychological factors in the irritable bowel syndrome. Eur J Med Res 2003; 8:549-556.

21   Riedl A, Schmidtmann M, Stengel A, Goebel M, Wisser AS, Klapp AS, Monnikes H. Somatic comorbidities of irritable bowel syndrome: A systematic analysis. J Psychosom Res 2008; 64:573-582.

22   Pimentel M, Chow EJ, Lin HC. Eradication of small intestinal bacterial overgrowth reduces symptoms of irritable bowel syndrome. Am J Gastroenterol 2000; 95(12):3503-3506.

23   Chadwick VS, Chen W, Shu D, Paulus B, Bethwaite P, Tie A, Wilson I. Activation of the mucosal immune system in irritable bowel syndrome. Gastroenterology 2002; 122(7):1778-1783.

24   Marshall JK, Thabane M, Garg AX, Clark W, Meddings J, Collins SM. Intestinal permeability in patients with irritable bowel syndrome after a waterborne outbreak of acute gastroenteritis in Walkerton, Ontario. Aliment Pharmacol Ther 2004; 20:1317-1322.

25   Atkinson W, Lockhart S, Whorwell PJ, Keevil B, Houghton LA. Altered 5-hydroxytryptamine signaling in patients with constipation- and diarrhea-predominant irritable bowel syndrome. Gastroenterology 2006; 130:34-43.

26   Lind CD. Motility disorders in the irritable bowel syndrome. Gastroenterol Clin North Am 1991; 20:279-95.

27   Delvaux M. Role of visceral sensitivity in the pathophysiology of irritable bowel syndrome. Gut 2002; 51S:i67-i71.

28   Marshall JK, Thabane M, Garg AX, Clark WF, Salvadori M, Collins SM. Incidence and epidemiology of irritable bowel syndrome after a large waterborne outbreak of bacterial dysentery. Gastroenterology 2006; 131:445-50.

29   Martinez-Martinez LA, Mora T, Fuentes-Iniestra M, Martinez-Lavin M. Sympathetic nervous system dysfunction in fibromyalgia, chronic fatigue syndrome, irritable bowel syndrome, and interstitial cystitis. J Clin Rheumatol 2014; 20:146-150.

30   Kalantar JS, Locke GR, Zinsmeister AR, Beighley CM, Talley NJ. Familial aggregation of irritable bowel syndrome: A prospective study. Gut 2003; 52:1703-1707.

31   Sainsbury A, Ford AC. Beyond fiber and antispasmodic agents. Ther Adv Gastroenterol 2011; 4:115-127.

32   Longstreth GF, Yao JF. Irritable bowel syndrome and surgery: a multivariable analysis. Gastroenterology 2004; 126:1665-1673.

33   Prior A, Whorwell PJ. Gynaecological consultation in patients with the irritable bowel syndrome. Gut 1989; 30:996-998.

34   Brandt LJ, Chey WD, Foxx-Orenstein AE, Schiller LR, Schoenfeld PS, Spiegel BM, Talley NJ, Quigley EM. An evidence-based position statement on the management of irritable bowel syndrome. Am J Gstroenterol 2009; 104:S1-35.

35   Ford AC, Chey WD, Talley NJ, Malhotra A, Spiegel BM, Moayyedi P. Yield of diagnostic tests for celiac disease in individuals with symptoms suggestive of irritable bowel syndrome: systematic review and meta-analysis. Arch Intern Med 2009; 13:169:651-658.

36   Stapel SO, Asero R, Ballmer-Weber BK, Knol EF, Strobel S, Vieths S, Kleine-Tebbe J. Testing for IgG4 against foods is not recommended as a diagnostic tool: EAACI Force Report. Allergy 2008; 63:793-796.

37   Ohman L, Lindmark AC, Isaksson S, Posserud I, Strid H, Sjovall H, Simren M. B-cell activation in patients with irritable bowel syndrome (IBS). Neurogastroenterol Motil 2009; 21:644-650.

38   Cremon C, Gargano L, Morsell-Labate AM, Santini D, Cogliandro RD, De Giorgio R, Stanghellini V, Corinaldesi R, Barbara G. Mucosal immune activation in irritable bowel syndrome: gender-dependence and association with digestive symptoms. Am J Gastroenterol. 2009; 104:392-400.

39   Laker MJ, Menzies IS. Increase in human intestinal permeability following ingestion of hypertonic solutions. J Physiol 1977; 265:881-894.

40 Tana C, Umesaki Y, Imaoka A, Handa T, Kanazawa M, Fukudo S. Altered profiles of intestinal microbiota and organic acids may be the origin of symptoms in irritable bowel syndrome. Neurogastroenterol Motil 2010; 22:512-519.

41 Philpott H, Nandurkar S, Lubel J, Gibson PR. Alternative investigations for irritable bowel syndrome. J Gastroenterol Hepatol 2013; 28:73-77.

42 Simren M, Stotzer PO. Use and abuse of hydrogen breath tests. Gut Mar 2006; 55:297-303.

43 Bijkerk CJ, de Wit NJ, Muris JW, Whorwell PJ, Knottnerus JA, Hoes AW. Soluble or insoluble fiber in irritable bowel syndrome in primary care? Randomised placebo controlled trial. BMJ [Internet]. [Cited 2009 Aug 27]; Available from: http://www.bmj.com/content/339/bmj.b3154.

44 Francis CY, Whorwell PJ. Bran and irritable bowel syndrome: time for reappraisal. Lancet 1994; 344:39-40.

45 Barclay L. Irritable Bowel Syndrome: New dietary guidelines. Medscape Medical News [Internet]; [cited 2012 May 18]. Available from: http://www.medscape.org/viewarticle/764083

46 Staudacher HM, Irving PM, Lomer MCE, Whelan K. Mechanisms and efficacy of dietary FODMAP restriction in IBS. Nat Rev Gastroenterol Hepatol 2014; 11:256-266.

47 The Low FODMAP Diet. Stanford Hospital & Clinics Digestive Health Center Nutrition Services. [Internet]; Available at: http://stanfordhealthcare.org/content/dam/SHC/for-patients-component/programs-Services/clinical-nutrition-services/Docs/pds-lowfodmapdiet.pdf

48   Yoon JS, Sohn W, Lee OY, Lee SP, Lee KN, Jun DW, Lee HL, Yoon BC, Choi HS, Chung WS, Seo JG. Effect of multispecies probiotics on irritable bowel syndrome. J Gastroenterol Hepatol 2014; 29:52-59.

49   O'Mahoney L, McCarthy J, Kelly P, Hurley G, Luo F, Chen K, O'Sullivan GC, Kiely B, Collins JK, Shanahan F, Quigley EM. Lactobacillus and bifidobacterium in irritable bowel syndrome: Symptom responses and relationship to cytokine profiles. Gastroenterology 2005; 128:541-551.

50   Verdu EF, Bercik P, Verma-Gandhu M, Huang XX, Blennerhassete P, Jackson W, Mao Y, Wang L, Rochat F, Collins SM. Specific probiotic therapy attenuates antibiotic induced visceral hypersensitivity in mice. Gut 2006; 55:182-190.

51   Mertz HR. Irritable Bowel Syndrome. N Engl J Med 2003; 349:2136-2146.

52   Spiller R, Aziz Q, Creed F, Emmanuel A, Houghton L, Hungin P, Jones R, Kumar D, Rubin G, Trudgill N, Whorwell P. Guidelines on the irritable bowel syndrome: mechanisms and practical management. Gut 2007; 56:1770-1798.

53   Sciarretta G, Fumo A, Mazzoni M, Malaguti P. Post-cholecystectomy diarrhea: evidence of bile acid malabsorption assessed by SeHCAT test. Am J Gastroenterol 1992; 87:1852-1854.

54   Irritable bowel syndrome. Mayo Clinic [Internet]; [cited 2008 December 1]. Available from: http://www.mayoclinic.org/diseases-conditions/irritable-bowel-syndrome/basics/definition/CON-20024578.

55   Ford AC, Talley NJ, Spiegel BMR, Foxx-Orenstein AE, Schiller L, Quigley EMM, Moayyedi P. Effect of fibre, antispasmodics, and peppermint oil in the treatment of irritable bowel syndrome: Systematic review and meta-analysis. British Journal of Medicine 2008:377:a2312.

56   National Center for Complementary and Alternative Medicine. Peppermint oil [Internet]. Available from: http://nccam.nih.gov/health/peppermintoil.

57   Difenoxin-atropine. [Internet]: Available at: http://www.webmd.com/drugs/2/drug-2313/difenoxin-atropine-oral/details.

58   Gorard DA, Healy JC, O'Donnell LJD, Farthing MJG. Inhibition of 5-hydroxytryptamine reuptake impairs human gallbladder emptying. Alimentary Pharmacology & Therapeutics 1994; 8:461-463.

59   Mayer EA, Bradesi S. Alosetron and irritable bowel syndrome. Expert Opin Pharmacother 2003:4:2089-2098.

60   Attar A, Lemann M, Ferguson A, Halphen M, Boutron M, Flourie B, Alix E, Salmeron M, Guillemot F, Chaussade S, Menard A, Moreau J, Naudin G, Barthet M. Comparison of a low dose polyethylene glycol electrolyte solution with lactulose for treatment of chronic constipation. Gut 1999; 44:226-230.

61   Camilleri M, Barucha AE, Ueno R, Burton D, Thomforde GM, Baxter K. Effect of a selective chloride channel activator, lubiprostone, on gastrointestinal transit, gastric sensory, and motor functions in healthy volunteers. Am J Physiol Gastrointest Liver Physiol 2006; 290:942-947.

62   Layer P, Stanghellini V. Linaclotide for the management of irritable bowel syndrome with constipation. Aliment Pharmacol Ther 2014; 39:371-384.

63   Trimble KC, Farouk R, Pryde A, Douglas S, Heading RC. Heightened visceral sensation in functional gastrointestinal disease is not site-specific. Evidence for a generalized disorder of gut sensitivity. Dig Dis Sci 1995; 40:1607-1613.

64   Gorard DA, Libby GW, Farthing MJ. Influence of antidepressants on whole gut orocaecal transit times in health and irritable bowel syndrome. Aliment Pharmacol Ther 1994; 8:159-166.

65   Drossman DA, Toner BB, Whitehead WE, Diamant NE, Dalton CB, Duncan S, Emmott S, Proffitt V, Akman D, Frusciante K, Le T, Meyer K, Bradshaw B, Mikula K, Morris CB, Blackman CJ, Hu Y, Hia H, Li JZ, Koch GG, Bangdiwala SI. Cognitive-behavioral therapy versus education and desipramine versus placebo for moderate to severe functional bowel disorders. Gastroenterology 2003; 125:19-31.

66   Saadi M, McCallum RW. Rifaximin in irritable bowel syndrome. Ther Adv Chronic Dis 2013; 4:71-75.

67   Bolen BB. IBS Management Guidelines 2009. What your doctor knows about treating IBS [Internet]; [cited 2009 January 22]. Available from: http://ibs.about.com/od/Treatmentofibs/a/IBSManagement.htm.

68   Pimentel M, Lembo A, Chey WD, Zakko S, Ringel Y, Yu J, Mareya SM, Shaw AL, Bortey E, Forbes WP. TARGET Study Group. Rifaximin therapy for patients with irritable bowel syndrome without constipation. N Engl J Med 2011; 364:22-32.

69   Low K, Hwang L, Hua J, Zhu A, Morales W, Pimentel M. A combination of rifaximin and neomycin is most effective in treating irritable bowel syndrome patients with methane on lactulose breath test. J Clin Gastroenterol 2010; 44:547-550.

70   Houghton LA, Fell C, Whorwell PJ, Jones I, Sudworth DP, Gale JD. Effect of second-generation α2δ ligand (pregabalin) on visceral sensation in hypersensitive patients with irritable bowel syndrome. Gut 2007; 56:1218-1225.

71   Hulisz D. The burden of illness of irritable bowel syndrome: current challenges and hope for the future. J Manag Care Pharm 2004; 10:299-309.

72   Drossman DA, Morris CB, Schneck S, Hu YJB, Norton NJ, Norton WF, Weinland S, Dalton C, Leserman J, Bangdiwala SI. International survey of patients with IBS: symptom features and their severity, health status, treatments, and risk taking to achieve clinical benefit. J Clin Gastroenterol. 2009; 43:541-550.

73   Ford AC, Moayyedi P. Meta-analysis: factors affecting placebo response rate in the irritable bowel syndrome. Alimentary Pharmacology & Therapeutics. 2010; 32:144-158.

74   Tornblom H, Lindberg G, Nyberg B, Veress B. Full-thickness biopsy of the jejunum reveals inflammation and enteric neuropathy in irritable bowel syndrome. Gastroenterology. 2002; 123:1972-1979.

75   Chadwick VS, Chen W, Shu D, Paulus B, Bethwaite P, Tie A, Wilson I. Activation of the mucosal immune system in irritable bowel syndrome. Gastroenterology. 2002; 122:1778-1783.

76 Collins SM. Is the irritable gut an inflamed gut? Scand J Gastroenterol 1992; 192(S):102-105.

77 Vergnolle N. Modulation of visceral pain and inflammation by protease-activated receptors. Br J Pharmacol 2004; 141:1264-1274.

78 Lind CD. Motility disorders in the irritable bowel syndrome. Gastroenterol Clin North Am 1991:20:279-295.

79 Isgar B, Harman M, Kaye MD, Whorwell PJ. Symptoms of irritable bowel syndrome in ulcerative colitis in remission. Gut 1983; 24:190-192.

80 Keohane J, O'Mahoney C, O'Mahoney L, O'Mahony S, Quigley EM, Shanahan F. Irritable bowel syndrome-type symptoms in patients with inflammatory bowel disease: a real association or reflection of occult inflammation? Am J Gastroenterol 2010; 1789-1794.

81 Thabane M, Kottachchi D, Marshall JK. Systematic review and meta-analysis: Incidence and prognosis of post-infectious irritable bowel syndrome. Aliment Pharmacol Ther 2007; 26:535-544.

82 Boyce JA, Arshad SH, Assa'ad A, Bahna SL, Beck LA, Burks AW, Jones SM, Sampson HA, Wood RA, Plaut M, Cooper SF, Fenton MJ ,Byrd-Bredbenner C, Camargo CA Jr, Eichenfield L, Furuta GT, Hanifin JM, Jones C, Kraft M, Levy BD, Lieberman P, Luccioli S, McCall KM, Schneider LC, Simon RA, Simons FE, Teach SJ, Yawn BP, Schwaninger JM. Guidelines for the diagnosis and management of food allergy. J Allergy Clin Immunol 2010; 126:S1-58.

83   Stierstorfer MB, Sha CT, Sasson M. Food patch testing for irritable bowel syndrome. J Am Acad Dermatol 2013 68:377-84.

84   Rietschel RL, Fowler JF Jr. Fisher's contact dermatitis. Hamilton, Ontario (Canada): BCDecker; 2008. p. 701-702.

85   Inadomi JM, Fennerty, MB, Bjorkman D. The economic impact of irritable bowel syndrome. Aliment Pharmacol Ther 2003:18:671-682.

86   Spergel JM, Brown-Whitehorn TF, Beausoleil JL, Franciosi J, Shuker M, Verma R, Liacouras CA. 14 years of eosinophilic esophagitis: clinical features and prognosis. J Pediatr Gastroenterol Nutr 2009; 48:30-36.

87   Spergel JM, Andrews T, Brown-Whitehorn TF, Beausoleil JL, Liacouras CA. Treatment of eosinophilic esophagitis with specific food elimination diet directed by a combination of skin prick and patch tests. Ann Allergy Asthma Immunol 2005; 95:336-343.

88   Leaky gut syndrome: what is it? WebMD [Internet]: Available at: http://www.webmd.com/digestive-disorders/features/leaky-gut-syndrome

89   Kiefer D, Ali-Akbarian. A brief evidence-based review of two gastrointestinal illnesses: irritable bowel and leaky gut syndromes. Alternative Therapies in Health and Medicine 2004; 10:22-30.

90   Catassi C, Bai J, Bonaz B, Bouma G, Calabro A, Carroccio A, Castillejo G, Ciacci C, Cristofori, F, Dolinsek J, Francavilla R, Elli L, Green P, Holtmeier W, Koehler P, Koletzko S, Meinhold C, Sanders D, Schumann M, Schuppan D, Ulrich R, Vecsei A, Volta U, Zevallos V, Sapone A, Fasano A. Non-celiac gluten sensitivity: The new frontier of gluten related disorders. Nutrients 2013; 5:3839-385.

About the Author

Michael Stierstorfer, M.D. is a board-certified dermatologist in North Wales and Philadelphia, Pennsylvania. He is the pioneer of the usefulness of food patch testing for IBS and IBS-like symptoms, and is the founder of East Penn Dermatology, P.C. and the IBS Centers for Advanced Food Allergy Testing, LLC. He specializes in medical, surgical and cosmetic dermatology.

Dr. Stierstorfer graduated with honors from Franklin & Marshall College and the Temple University School of Medicine. He completed his Internal Medicine internship and Dermatology residency at the Dartmouth-Hitchcock Medical Center, where he served as Chief Resident. He is a Clinical Associate Professor of Dermatology at the University of Pennsylvania School of Medicine, where he supervises Dermatology residents in training and was awarded a Faculty Teaching Award in 2008.

He is a member of the American Academy of Dermatology, the Pennsylvania Academy of Dermatology and Dermatological Surgery, and the Philadelphia Dermatological Society. He has published in a number of peer-reviewed dermatology journals and is a clinical investigator independently and with the Dermatology Clinical Effectiveness Research Network (DCERN) and a participant in the Major League Baseball Skin Cancer Screening and Awareness Program.

Made in the USA
Middletown, DE
06 February 2018